12 Lead EKG
in about an hour!

JOSEPH BARNES, EMTP, CCEMTP, CCPP, PICCP, EMSI, IC

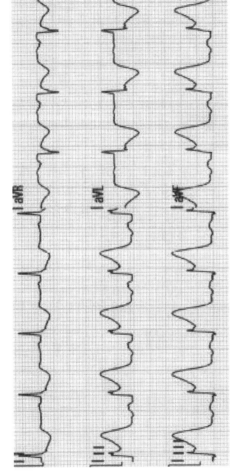

Copyright 2013. Joseph Barnes, 𝕸𝖊𝖉𝖎𝖈𝖘𝖒𝖎𝖙𝖍 𝖘𝖊𝖗𝖎𝖊𝖘

12 Lead EKG in about an hour!

All rights reserved.

Information from this book may not be used all or in part without the written consent of the Joseph Barnes

Dedication

This book and all books in the **Medicsmith Series** are dedicated to Esmeralda Barnes and will become the sole property of Esmeralda Barnes upon death or disability of Joseph Barnes.

Table of Contents

Introduction		5
Chapter 1	The EKG	8
Chapter 2	It is What it is	10
Chapter 3	Do Not Skip Ahead	14
Chapter 4	Bundle Branch Blocks	35
Chapter 5	What Can We See	40
Practice Rhythms		46
Reference		81
Critical Care Paramedic Practitioner		82

T

his book started over a decade ago as a training series during a Medical Flight from the Mayo Clinic to Kuwait City, Kuwait with a vented cardiac patient. I was with an extremely talented nurse who had successfully navigated her way around learning 12 Lead EKG's. Along with several medics I had known over the years, the 12 Lead EKG was intimidating and a foreign language. On the 13 hour return flight I wrote this course and shared with her. When we landed back in New York she was bangin' thru 12 Lead tracings and having a great time. *You will be no different*.

In the Army back in the early 90's I was asked to teach in a new program called the Combat Lifesavers training. I was preparing for the class with the curriculum in hand when the Captain over the program told me, "Now remember to write the class and lectures at the 8th grade level so all of the soldiers will understand the information." I was dumbfounded at the thought of teaching IV therapy, Anatomy and Physiology, not to mention the treatment of sucking chest wounds, all at an 8th grade comprehension level. However after way more time than it should have taken, I had a class. I found that I enjoyed teaching at that level so much I have carried that concept with me for the rest of my carrier.

Some may argue that classes taught in that mindset, especially those involving medicine and treatments could not possible cover all that is required. To those I say, this style of learning may not be for you. But for the thousands of students I have taught over the years it works.

While working as a Hurricane responder at Katrina in Louisiana I was challenged by an EMS Director. This individual was confident that a systematic approached to cardiac evaluation at the 8th grade level was not possible. So, with 4 of that Directors paramedics, 1 nurse, and the cleaning lady of the church where we were being housed for the hurricane I gave the lecture. At the end of the class, everyone at the table was able to pass the American Heart ACLS 12 Lead Interpretation test; including the cleaning lady.

Now the disclaimer:

In this course I'm not looking to make you a Doctor, or a master clinician. My goal is basic recognition of 12 Lead EKG tracings as it relates to identifying cardiac injury.

With that said here are the rules for using this course:

1. For total comprehension, follow the exercises completely as written.
2. Do NOT jump ahead.
3. Remember rule 1.

4. Remember rule 2.
5. See rule number 1.

Trust me when I tell you to follow the program page by page. Some of the exercises may seem rudimentary for some of you big brains. But if you had already nailed 12 Leads you would not have bought this book.

6. This is not an EKG book. I will not be teaching you to read basic EKG tracings. I will do a quick review to refresh your memory, but you should already have a basic understanding of EKG's to navigate this program.
7. Relax and have fun. About halfway thru the book you will think I'm crazy but stick out the hour and your opinion may change.
8. In this book I use the word ASS. If this offends you I would apologize but it would not be sincere. It is what it is.
9. In this book I use the word Habeeb. This is what my friend and counterpart in Kuwait called me. So to anyone who gets offended by the use of this word I would say, "The word means friend, and in the training I am referring to myself!"

Enough Rules!

Chapter 1

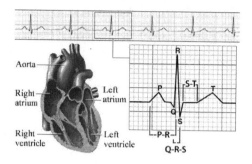

The EKG

The EKG is an instrument used to measure electricity. Get out of your head that it measures anything the heart is physically doing. It merely records the passage of electrical impulses along a predetermined pathway to create motion in an object.

The tracing that is created on a graphed piece of paper is divided into identifiable waves: P, Q, R, S, and T. There is no great science in the determining to name these waves as such. It was simply the letters in the alphabet in sequence that, at the time were not allocated to something else. BRILLIANT!

The "P" wave, and upward sloping small wave comes first on the base line and for all intensive purposes should be 3 to 5 small boxes away from the next wave on the graph. It relates to the atrial side of the heart and is sometimes hard to identify in some accelerated rhythms.

The "Q" wave not always present on an EKG is usually a downward stroke or notch. In some cases it signifies injury to the heart, AS LONG AS IT IS AT LEAST 1/3RD THE SIZE OF THE QRS COMPLEX.

The "RS" wave combination is the larger of the waves on the base line and show the actual contraction of the ventricular side of the heart.

The "T" is the last upward sloping wave on the base line and identifies the heart at rest. It is also a marker for ischemia, or lack of Oxygen in the heart, should the "T" wave become inverted. The "T" wave can also relate to serum Potassium levels.

The spaces between the waves are referred to as intervals.

In most training programs Paramedics are taught to read Lead II. In this class I call that the "Paramedic Lead".

That completes the refresher for the EKG. It was very simplistic and not meant to teach you to read and 3 Lead or 4 Lead EKG tracing.

Now let's do 12 Leads!

Chapter 2

It Is What It Is

There she is, The Mustang GT. A highly tuned, master of speed and power; American muscle. I want you to think of the heart just like this mustang…. Now follow me here. If I asked you to show me the grill you would most easily point out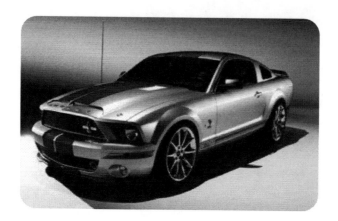

There is no argument in that answer. In

the same fashion, if I asked you to point out the rear driver side tire, I'm sure there is not a one of us who could not find where to go:

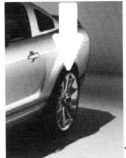 Yep there it is….

We have confidence in identifying the different sides of a vehicle because we can touch it, we have experience in driving or riding in cars. But when it comes to the heart, the physical piece of meat it gets confusing. What we must try to understand that as it relates to a 12 Lead EKG and the damage that we are looking for when we run a 12 lead EKG, it should be the same as identifying the different sides of a car.

The heart has sides or planes, identified as:

Anterior Side – we will identify with an "A".

Posterior Side – we will identify with a "P".

Inferior Side – we will identify with an "I".

Septal Area – we will identify with an "S".

Lateral (HIGH) Side – identified as "HL".

Lateral (LOW) Side – identified as "L".

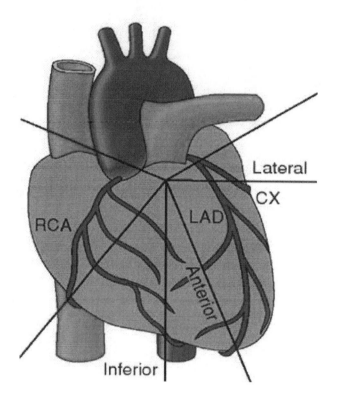

Obviously from this view you cannot see the posterior section or the septal section but just as with the mustang you know it is there. We have the technology to look at the Posterior view with the EKG with a Posterior EKG or 15 Lead EKG.

The heart sits in the chest just off center or midline and to view the electrical activity in the heart for a 12 lead we place 10 electrodes on the chest and extremities, as such:

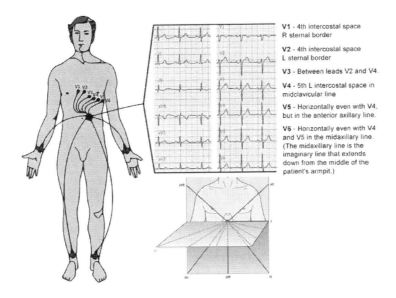

There is some discussion on the limb leads, using the shoulder verses the wrist, the sides of the lower torso verses the legs. For the most part EKG machines now display a diagram for placement. It is best to follow the diagram as drawn for the machine you are operating.

It should be understood that an EKG does not measure all of the electrical activity in the heart at the same time. By that I mean we know that there are electrical impulses happening in the heart in areas away from our placement of the electrodes. Our 12 Lead is looking at a specific electrical pathway from whatever view we chose to be monitoring.

Chapter 3

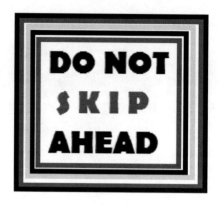

"EXERCISES"

Remember rule #1, and stay with me!!!

1. Gather a handful of blank paper, a ruler (optional), different color pens or pencils, and some room to do some art work.

Here we go---

Exercise 1:

The 12 Lead EKG printed has 12 individual block sections.

On a blank piece of paper or the space below, Draw a 12 Lead EKG as follows:

Exercise 2:

On the second sheet of paper or the space below, please write the following sentence 15 times: (exactly as written)

ALL ASSes In Iraq Including Little Habeeb are a Little Harry.

Exercise 3:

In another sheet of paper or the space below, draw the 12 Lead Diagram. In the first box, starting at the upper left corner, moving DOWN, identify the first 3 boxes as follows:

I			
II			
III			

Exercise 4:

The next set of boxes on the 12 Lead Diagram refer to the AV leads: AVR, AVL, AVF. Don't let that intimidate you, it simply means:

- AtrioVenticular Right (AVR)
- AtrioVenticular Left (AVL)
- AtriVenticular Foot (AVF)

On a new sheet of paper, or the space below, draw the 12 Lead Diagram, as follows:

I	AVR		
II	AVL		
III	AVF		

Exercise 5:

On a new sheet of paper, or the space below, draw the 12 Lead Diagram and identify the next 3 boxes as our first set of "V" leads:

I	AVR	V1	
II	AVL	V2	
III	AVF	V3	

Exercise 6:

On a new sheet of paper, or the space below, draw the 12 Lead Diagram and complete the identification with the last "V" leads.

I	AVR	V1	V4
II	AVL	V2	V5
III	AVF	V3	V6

Exercise 7:

On a new sheet of paper, or the space below, redraw the 12 Lead Diagram from Exercise 6 and circle II and AVR.

I	(AVR)	V1	V4
(II)	AVL	V2	V5
III	AVF	V3	V6

Brain *FOOOOOD*: (CHECK PLACEMENT) On a 12 Lead EKG the AVR Lead and Lead II are anatomical opposites. Lead II or the "Paramedic Lead" is what we are accustom to looking at in an EKG, but to make sure our placement is accurate for a 12 Lead, AVR should be similar or the same as Lead II, just upside down. The better the placement, the more accurate the mirrored image.

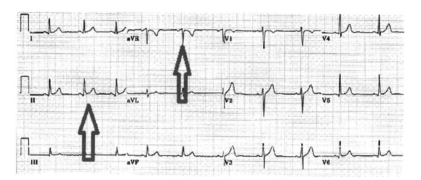

See how Lead II is the inverse of AVR.

Exercise 8:

On a new sheet of paper, draw the 12 Lead diagram as you did in Exercise 6. Then add in your best attempt to draw a Normal Sinus Rhythm in Lead II and an upside down version in AVR.

Exercise 9:

In Exercise 2 you had to write:

ALL ASSes In Iraq Including Little Habeeb are a Little Harry.

Now let's put into play. This sentence will identify all of the planes of the heart, anterior, inferior, septal, lateral, and high lateral.

On a new sheet of paper draw the 12 Lead Diagram from Exercise 6.

Next, starting on the Right side this time place the word ALL in the following boxes.

I	AVR	V1	V4	A
II	AVL	V2	V5	L
III	AVF	V3	V6	L

Remember the "A" stands for Anterior and the "L" stands for Lateral.

Exercise 10:

On a new sheet of paper, or on the space below, draw the 12 Lead Diagram from Exercise 9 and add the word ASSes as follows:

I	AVR	V1	S e S V4	A
II	AVL	V2	S V5	L
III	AVF	V3	A V6	L

Remember the "S" stands for Septal.

Exercise 11:

On a new sheet of paper, or on the space below, draw the Diagram from Exercise 10 and add the phrase "In Iraq Including" to the following boxes as follows:

				S e		
I		AVR		V1	S V4	A
II	I	AVL		V2	S V5	L
III	I	AVF	I	V3	A V6	L

Remember the "I" stands for Inferior.

Exercise 12:

On a new sheet of paper, or in the space below, draw the 12 Lead Diagram for Exercise 11. Add the final words of the sentence, "Little Harry".

						S e			A
I		HL	AVR		V1		S	V4	
II		I	AVL	HL	V2		S	V5	L
III		I	AVF	I	V3		A	V6	L

Exercise 13:

On a new sheet a paper, or in the space below draw the 12 Lead Diagram from Exercise 1 and label all the PLANES OF THE HEART.

I　　　　HL	AVR	V1　　　　S	V4　　　　A
HIGH LATERAL	(CHECK LEAD)	SEPTAL	ANTERIOR
II　　　　I	AVL　　　HL	V2　　　　S	V5　　　　L
INFERIOR	HIGH LATERAL	SEPTAL	LOW LATERAL
III　　　　I	AVF　　　I	V3　　　　A	V6　　　　L
INFERIOR	INFERIOR	ANTERIOR	LOW LATERAL

Color Diagram Chart

No we understand how to identify the sections of the 12 Lead and how they relate to the planes of the heat.

- You should remember from you basic EKG class that Wide is bad, and "ST" elevation in bad.
- You should remember that flattening or inverting of the "T" wave illustrates Ischemia.
- In 12 Lead EKG the term CONTIGUOUS refers to Leads on the same plane of the heart. To identify injury, you must have changes from NSR in 2 or more Leads from the same plane of the Heart.

Let's try an easy one…………..

- ✓ First check Lead placement by comparing Lead II to AVR. They should be anatomical opposites.
- ✓ Notice that Lead II has an upward stroke and AVR has a downward stroke.
- ✓ They are opposite and immediately we can tell there is something wrong.

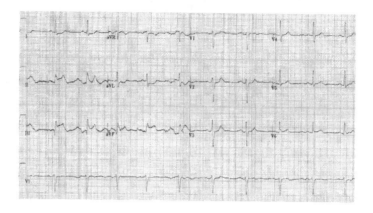

- ✓ Next, label the 12 Lead with the sentence we learned from Exercise 2

"ALL ASSes In Iraq Including Little Habeeb are a Little Harry."

Your 12 Lead should look like this:

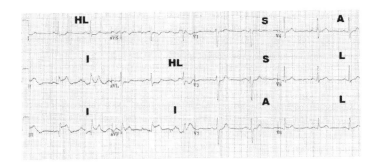

"ALL ASSes In Iraq Including Little Habeeb are a Little Harry."

✓ Now circle with a red pen everything that is wide or a "ST" elevation, or any "Q" wave that is greater than 1/3 the size of the "RS" complex.

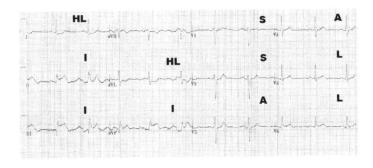

Your 12 Lead should look like this:

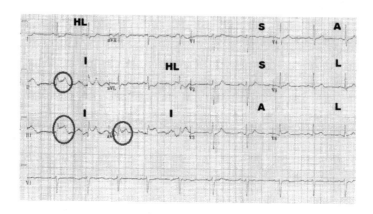

Now read the CIRCLES out loud.

This patient has an _____ wall MI.

(Inferior)

FOR EVERY 12 LEAD YOU WILL LABEL THE BOXES FROM RIGHT TO LEFT UTILIZING OR MEMORY SENTENCE.

***SAY IT OUT LOUD AS YOU LABEL THE BOXES.

*****LET YOURSELF HEAR THE MEMORY SENTENCE AS YOU WRITE IT DOWN.

Let's do another⟶ ⟶ ⟶ ⟶ ⟶

This time follow the order on your own:

1. Look for placement.
2. Label the boxes.
3. Circle any damage you see.
4. Read the EKG

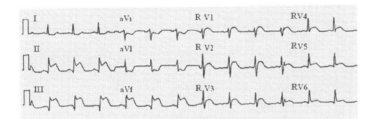

Write the diagnosis below:

_____

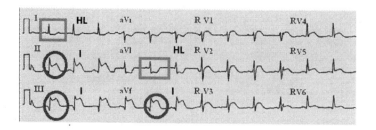

Diagnosis:

Acute Inferior Wall MI

with

Lateral ST Depression.

> The "ST" depression tells us the high lateral side of the heart is experiencing _____.
> **(Ischemia)**

If there had been damage in the Lateral Leads you would have joined Inferior & Lateral.

The patient would be experiencing an Inferolateral Wall MI.

Chapter 4

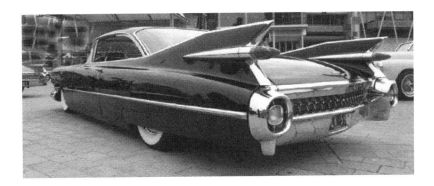

Bundle Branch Blocks

I want to take you on a trip, and you drivin'. This 1959 Caddy in the picture is our ride. Check out those BIG, WIDE fins.

So we are on our trip riding thru some small Texas town. Stick your arms out in front of you and grab the steering wheel….NO KIDDING…Get your arms up.

> *We identify Bundle Branch Blocks in Lead V1.*
>
> *Forget the old "Rabbit Ears" thing; it's wrong over 70% of the time.*
>
> *Your write a Bundle Branch Block either LBBB for Left or RBBB for Right.*

Now here comes a **LEFT** turn so reach down and push the turn signal **DOWN** and make a **BIG, WIDE** Left turn onto the downtown square. Let's just ride around the square a few times.

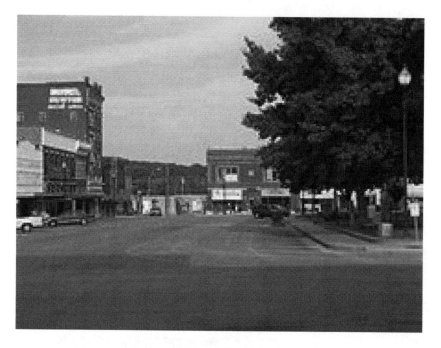

That's enough. Now make a **RIGHT** turn up there at the corner. Reach down and flip that turn signal **UP** and make a **BIG, RIGHT** hand turn off the square. What a great day for a ride!

Now for the next few minutes just talk yourself thru that drive again. Don't forget that you have to use your turn signal and make big, wide turns to get that Caddy around the corner without hitting anything.

● ● ●

Now let's put that drive down on a 12 Lead EKG. We look at V1 to find Bundle Branch Blocks (BBB).

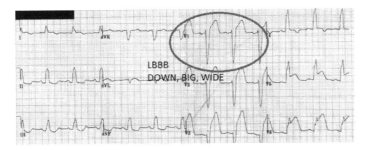

Left Bundle Branch Block

Just like driving our BIG car. TO make a left turn you must push the turn signal DOWN, and make a BIG, WIDE turn. Notice the "QRS" complex; Downward, Big, and Wide just like that Left turn in the Caddy.

As you are a keen student you probable noticed there is some damage in this 12 Lead so Label it out (SPEAKING OUT LOUD), then identify the injury and any Ischemia you may see.

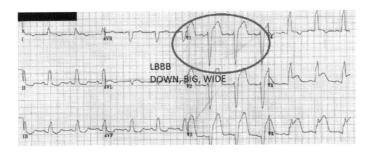

Diagnosis:

_____.

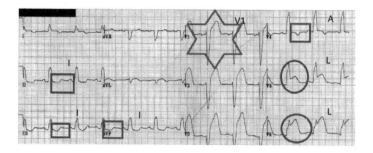

Lateral Wall MI with Inferior Ischemia in the presence of a Left Bundle Branch Block.

Back in the Caddy.

So we are on our trip (again) riding thru that small Texas town. Stick your arms out in front of you and grab the steering wheel….NO KIDDING…Get your arms up. ..Now make a **RIGHT** turn up there at the corner. Reach down and flip that turn signal **UP** and make a **BIG, RIGHT** hand turn off the square. What a great day for a ride!

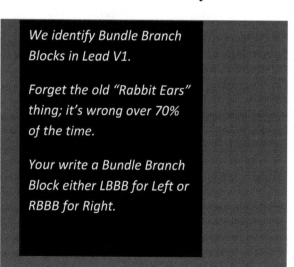

We identify Bundle Branch Blocks in Lead V1.

Forget the old "Rabbit Ears" thing; it's wrong over 70% of the time.

Your write a Bundle Branch Block either LBBB for Left or RBBB for Right.

Now for the next few minutes just talk yourself thru that drive again. Don't forget that you have to use your turn signal and make big, wide turns to get that Caddy around the corner without hitting anything.

Now let's put that drive down on a 12 Lead EKG. Remember we look at V1 to find Bundle Branch Blocks (BBB). Notice the "QRS" complex; Upward, Big, and Wide just like that Right turn in the Caddy

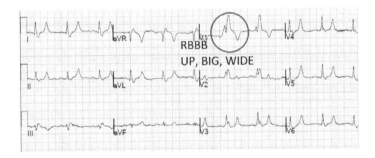

Right Bundle Branch Block

"QRS" Complex is UP, Big, and Wide.

Brain *FOOOOD*: Often in a significant Inferior cardiac incident a Bundle Branch Block will be found, depending on the location of the injury.

***There is something interesting going on in this 12 Lead. Notice that the "T" wave is elevated throughout. We know from Basic EKG that an elevated "T" wave could identify elevated Potassium levels. Always treat the patient not the EKG.

Chapter 5

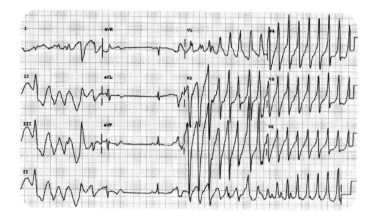

What Can We SEE

I was fortunate enough to spend more than a dozen years under some of the most impressive doctors in the business; to include Dr. Red Duke and members of the Red Team. To their credit and pacience, medics like me actually learned something. One day I remember, years ago when Mark McGuire, the "Big Mac" of professional baseball fame came into one of those ER's I was working. One of the other medics was the mother of McGuire's high school friend and he was there just to get a hug from her. Nice guy!

As he was leaving one of the patients popped off about "No man is worth what that guy is getting paid, just like these greedy Doctors". In an earlier part of my life I might have agreed with the patient. But I can remember thinking about all those Doc's who spent time with not just the patients, but me and the other Allied Health Professionals to share what they learned. So for what it's worth here is some of the wisdom these fantastic individuals shared with me. And for the record….they were worth every penny they were paid.

A special thanks to the Doctors that built me.

● ● ●

Left Ventricular Hypertrophy (LVH)

If a patient spends years and years suffering from Hypertension, the ventricles, just like any other muscle gain mass. Along with mass they can gain strength in the contraction; constantly fighting against the vascular resistance.

Over the years I have run thousands of 12 Leads, and with few exceptions, if LVH was present they had a history of LVH. After a while you stop asking if they have a history of HTN, you ask them how long have they had HTN.

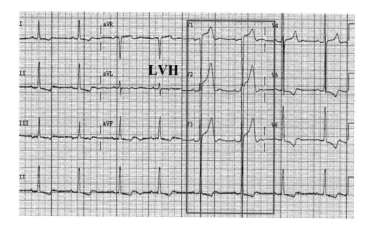

What else do you see?

Pulmonary Embolism

In the 25 or so years working patients I've had countless patients with PE's. These patients that we got back to the hospital in time complained of similar problems:

1. Chest Pain
2. Increased Pain with Inspiration
3. Tachycardia
4. V1, V2, V3 changes

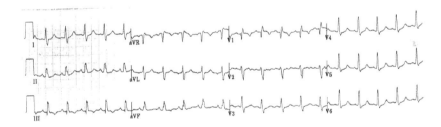

The chest pain, as much as the decreased oxygen is what is responsible for the tachycardia, changes in V1, V2, V3 relate to place and view of the heart.

RIGHT SIDED MI

In some patients there is good cause to check for what is referred to as a Right Sided MI. In the back of the ambulance with a patient time is important. Therefore if you suspect that your patient may have suffered a Right Sided MI due to ectopy in V4, V5, V6, move V4 from under the left nipple and place below the right nipple and run the test again.

Check V4 for the characteristic tracings associated with a cardiac event.

A little warning:

Sometimes on a Right Sided MI the size of the tracing may appear small so get out those glasses.

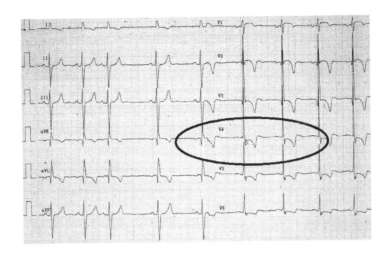

Don't Trust the Computer Interpretation

All computers eventually fail. That being said a lot of factors can affect the way the computer in the 12 Lead machines sees the EKG. Keep that in mind.

I was taught by ever great ER Doc I ever worked with to never look at the Computer Interpretation until you have made your own interpretation. To add to that, I was taught by a couple Cardiologists over the years, "only look at the Computer Interpretation if you want a good laugh."

PRACTICE

Along with each of these EKG's is the Interpretation.

- Take your time.
- Work the memory sentence.
- Label the 12 lead
- Name out loud the EKG.
- Don't over read the EKG

- Don't cheat.

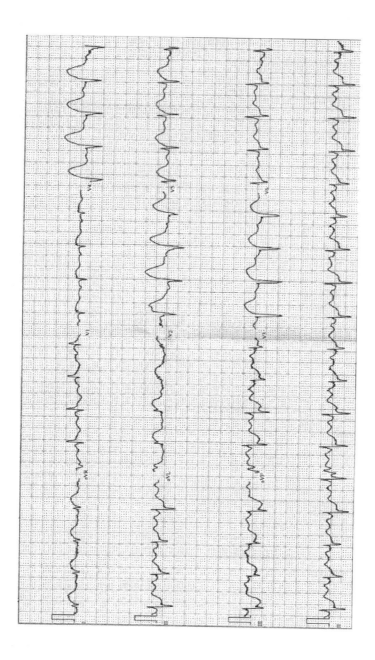

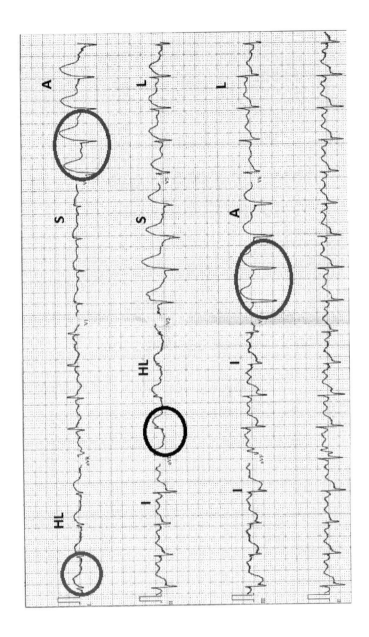

Anteriolateral Wall MI

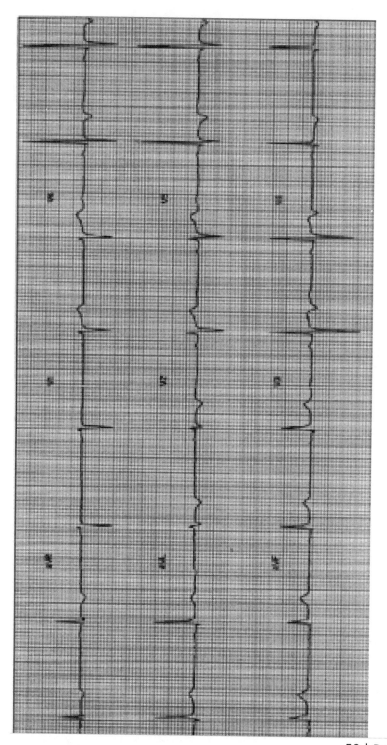

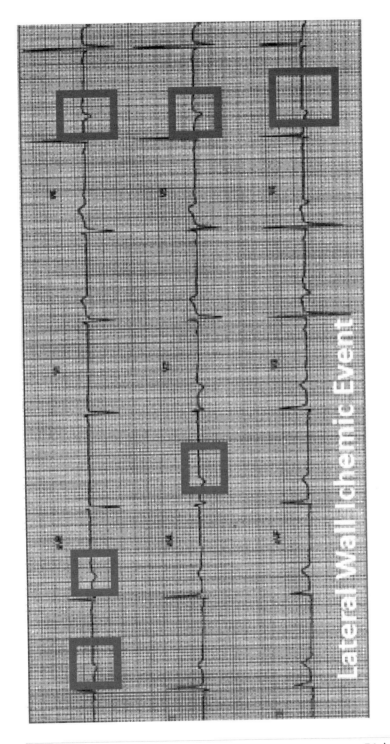

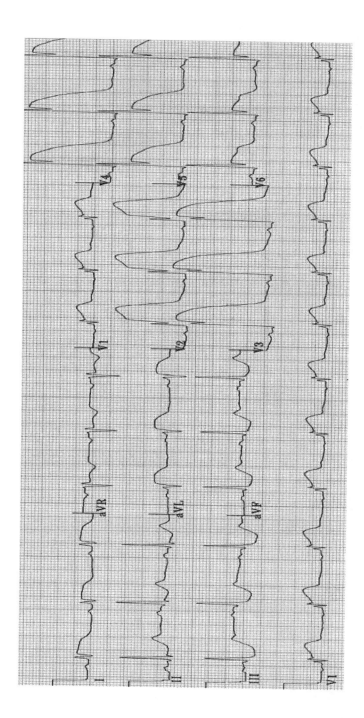

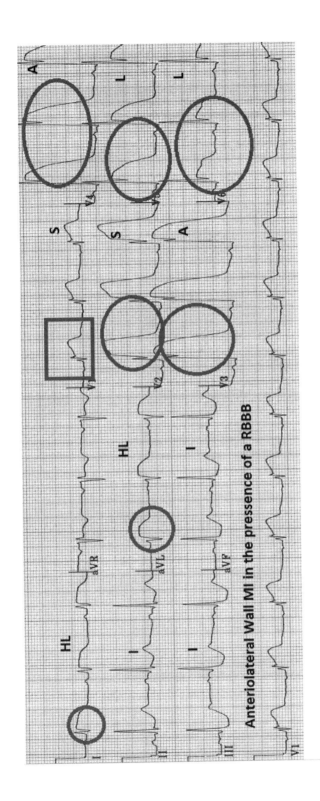

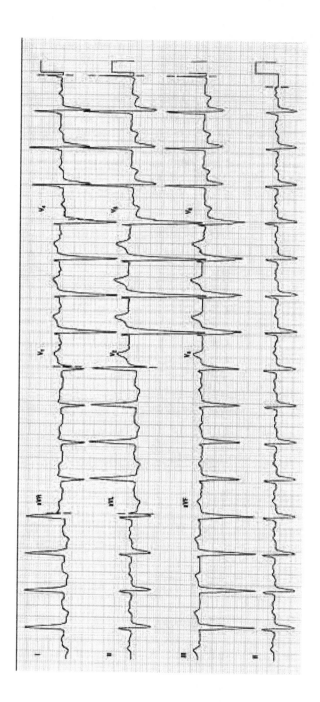

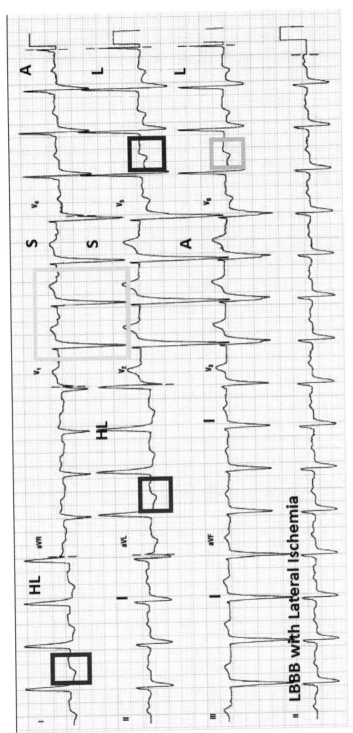

LBBB with Lateral Ischemia

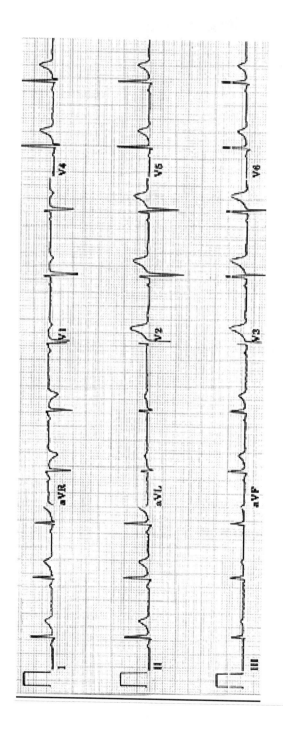

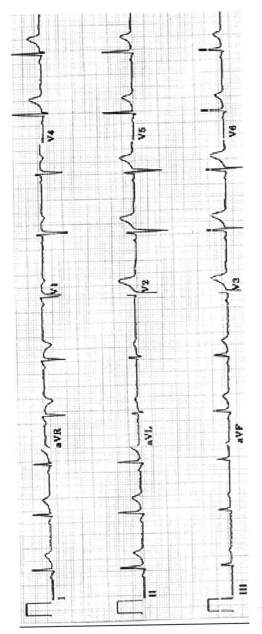

NSR

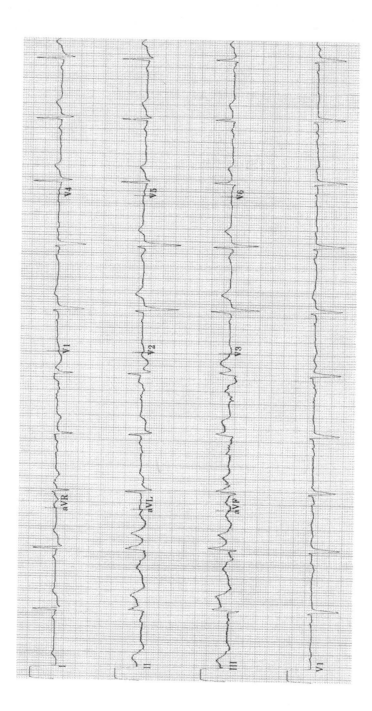

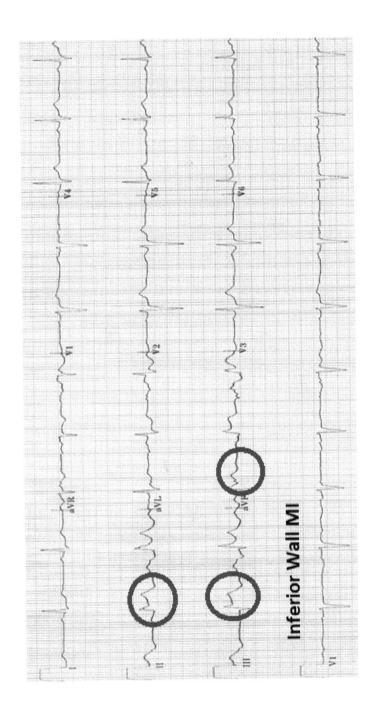

Inferior Wall MI

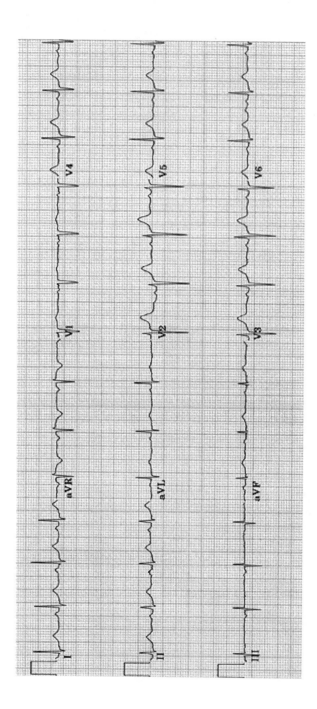

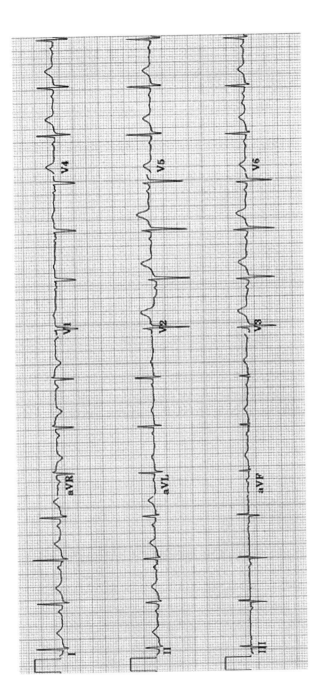

Sinus Rhythm

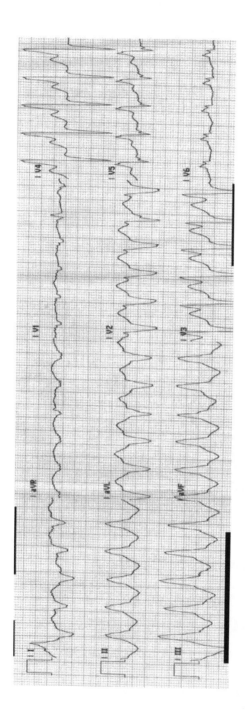

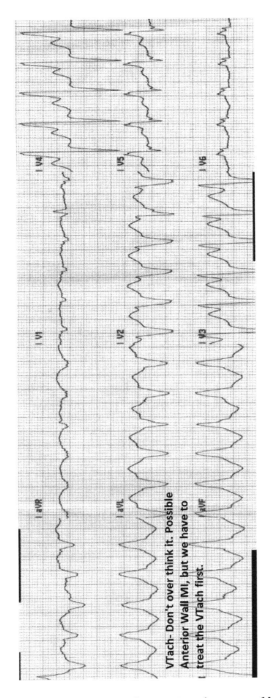

Wide Complex Tachycardia

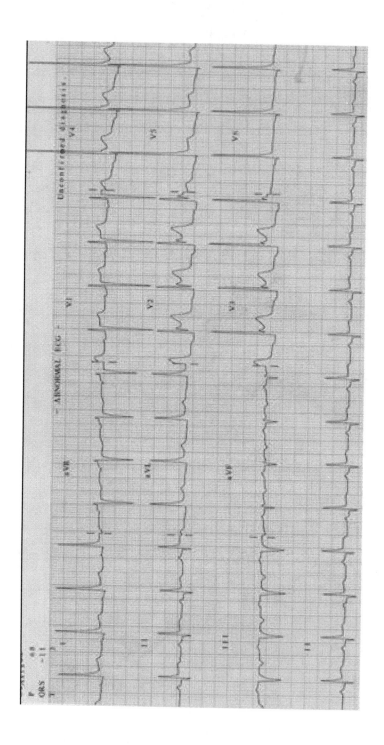

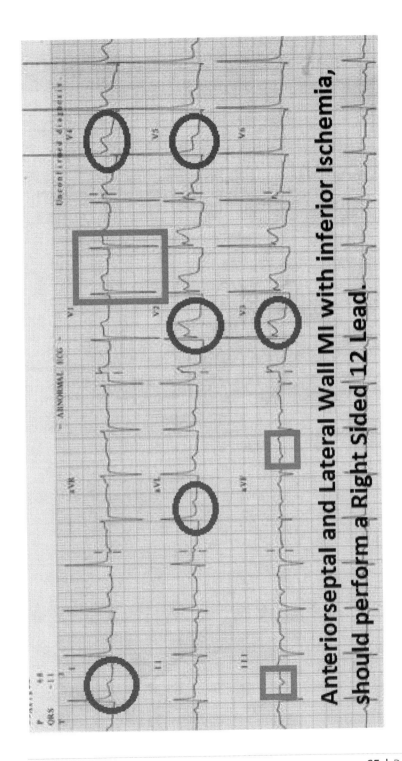

Anteriorseptal and Lateral Wall MI with inferior Ischemia, should perform a Right Sided 12 Lead.

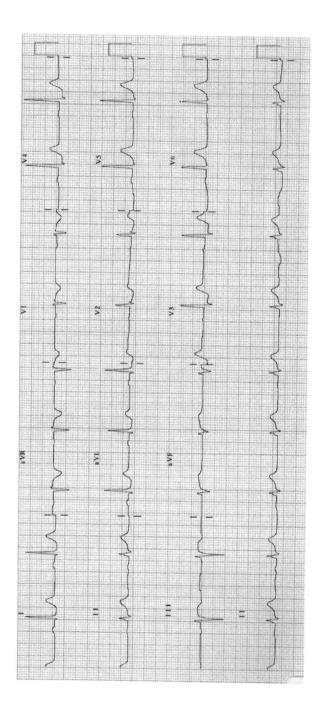

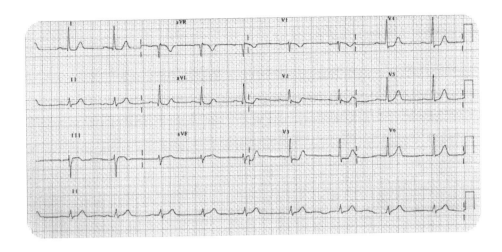

In patients presenting with ischemic symptoms, horizontal ST depression in leads V1-3 consider a posterior MI. As the posterior view cannot be seen in the standard 12-lead ECG, WHEN changes are visualized in leads V1-3 run a Posterior EKG by moving V4 (V7) to posterior axillary line of the base of the scapula, V5 (V8) base of the mid scapular in line with V4 (V7), V6 (V9) to the left of the spine on the same horizontal plane as the other leads. Run the 12 Lead again.

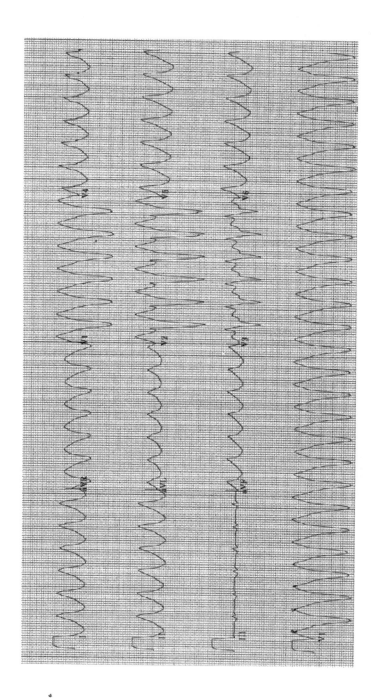

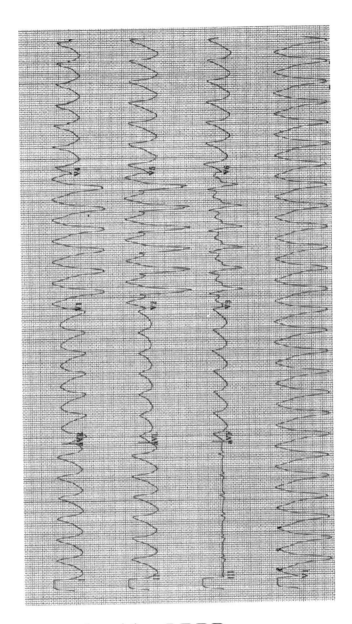

V-Tach with a LBBB

70 | Page

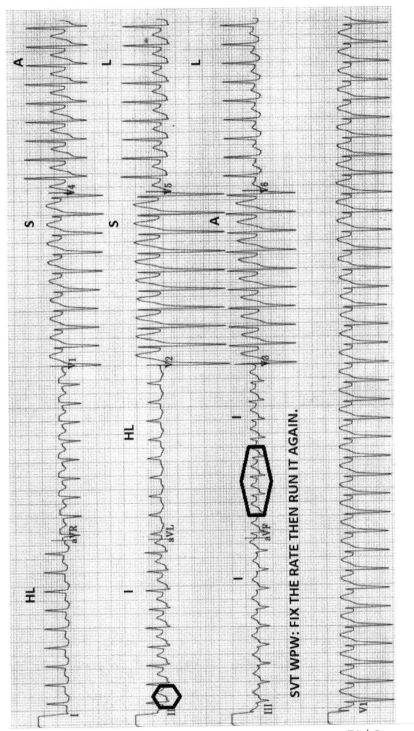

SVT WPW: FIX THE RATE THEN RUN IT AGAIN.

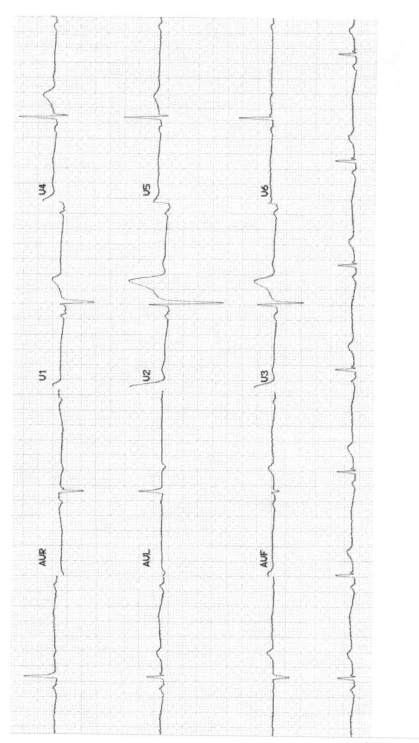

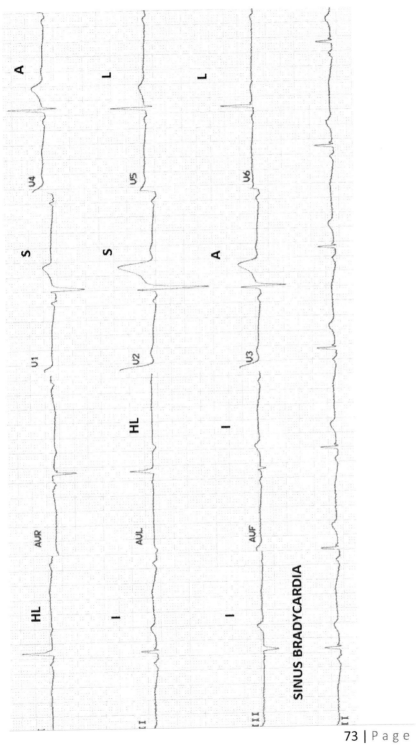

SINUS BRADYCARDIA

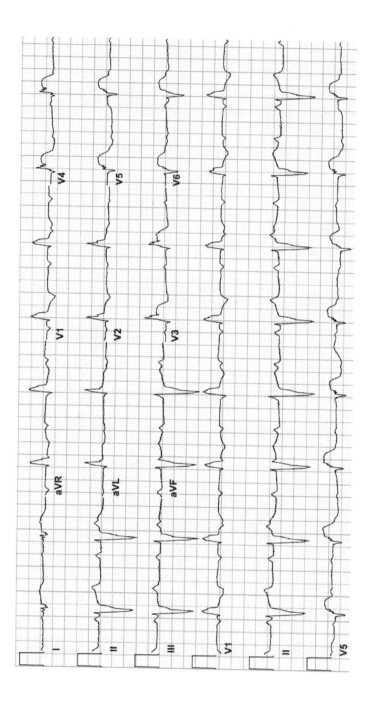

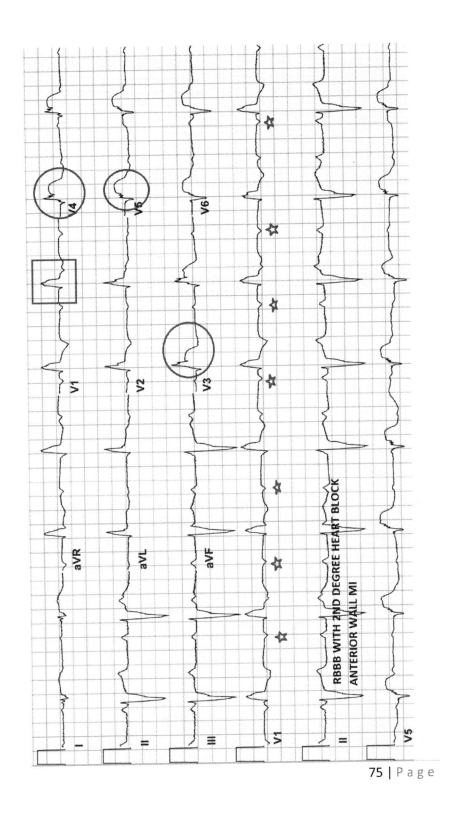

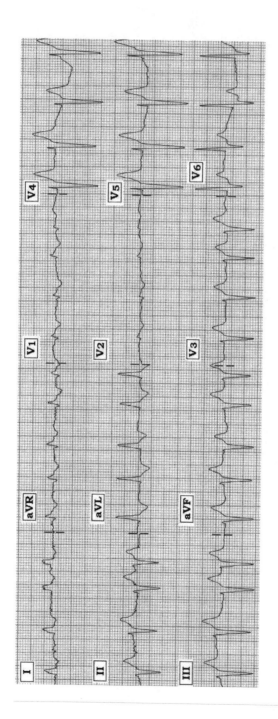

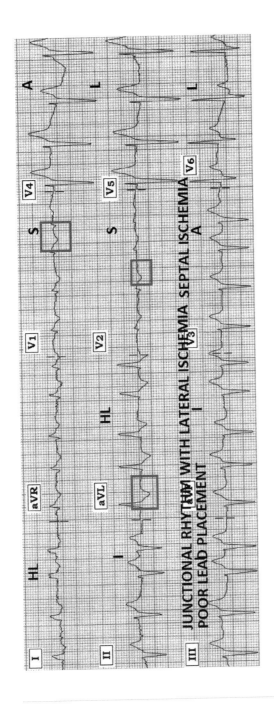

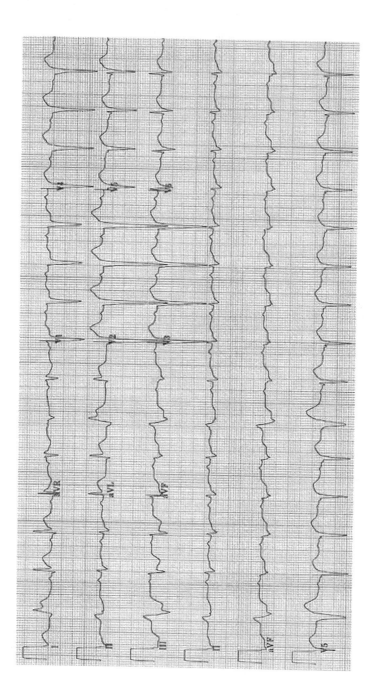

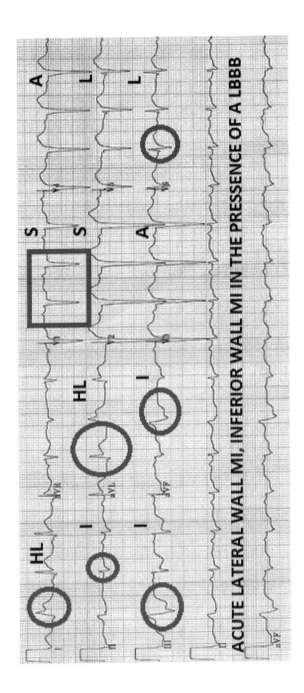

ACUTE LATERAL WALL MI, INFERIOR WALL MI IN THE PRESSENCE OF A LBBB

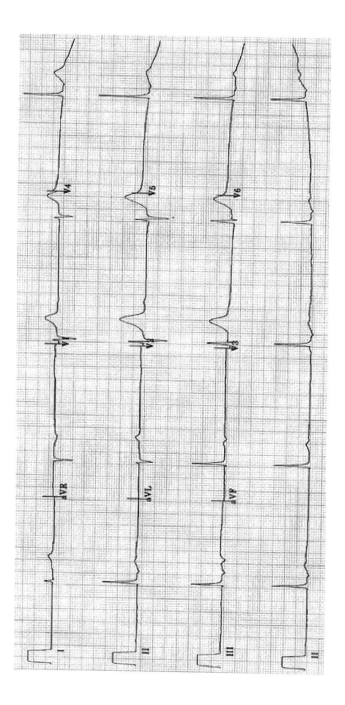

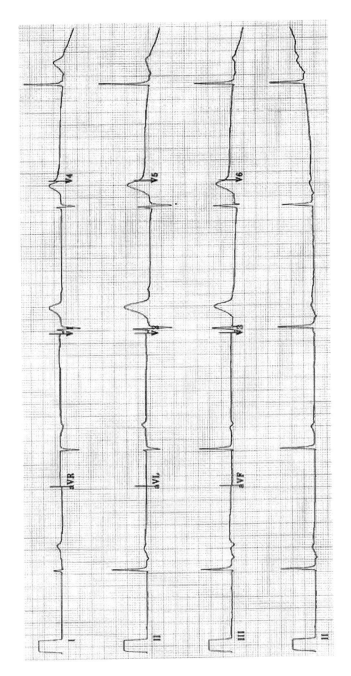

BRADYCARDIA

Reference

Drew, B.J., Krucoff, M.W. and the ST-Segment Monitoring Practice Guideline International Working Group (1999). Multilead ST-segment monitoring in patients with acute coronary syndromes: A consensus statement for healthcare professionals. American Journal of Critical Care, 8, 372-388.

Mizutani, M., Freedman, S.B., Barns, E., Ogasawara, S., Bailey, B.P. and Beinstein, L. (1990). ST Monitoring for myocardial Ischemia during and after coronary angioplasty. American Journal of Cardiology, 66(4), 389-393.

Stewart, R.B., Bardy, G.H. and Greene, L.H.(1986). Wide complex tachycardia: Misdiagnosis and outcomes after emergent therapy. Annals of Internal Medicine, 104, 766-771.

Wellens, J.J., Frits, W.H. and Lie, K.I. (1978). The value of the electrocardiogram in the differential diagnosis of a tachycardia with a widened QRS complex. The American Journal of Medicine, 64, 27-33.

Critical Care Paramedic Practitioner

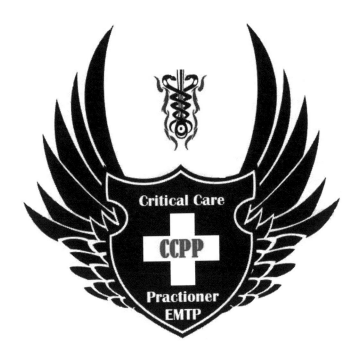

For Information on becoming a

Critical Care Paramedic Practitioner

OR to become an Instructor:

www.BarnesSouthwesternIT.com

Barnes Technical Institute is the ONLY AUTHORIZED SITE DISTROBUTION CENTER for the Critical Care Paramedic Practitioner certification and program.

Please report violations to the web address provided.

ALL EKG TRACINGS IN THIS SERIES HAVE BEEN VIEWED AND DIAGNOSED BY A LICENSE PHYSICIAN.

Made in the USA
Middletown, DE
23 February 2024

50204504R00049